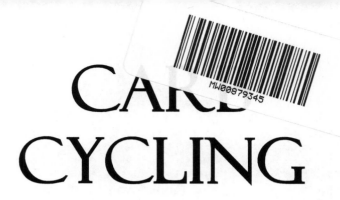

CARB CYCLING

The Recipe And Diet Book - Living Healthy And Fit Through Carb Cycling

INTRODUCTION

I want to thank and congratulate you for downloading the book *"Carb Cycling: Everything you need to know About Carb Cycling."*

This book contains proven steps and strategies on how to lose weight, burn fat and build muscle using the carb cycling diet. The carb cycling diet is very useful, as it will help you lose weight, gain muscle, and it will also restore your general body health and make you feel good. The diet is a popular known food diet which basically entails the switching of high carb and low carb days. It requires commitment and follow a specific plan, but the best thing about it is that it has cheat meals.

If you have been stressed about your weight or you want to gain muscle now, then this is the right book for you. It gives you a deeper understanding of carb cycling; starting with the basics, carb cycling program, shopping list, and meal plans. It also explains how exactly it will help you, as well as providing you with some high carb and low carb recipes. Much more will be discovered as you go through each chapter and you will find this dieting strategy to be very effective.

Our health is always a main concern and it is important that you learn and understand that along with helping you lose weight, the carb cycling diet is also one of the best ways to improve your overall health.

CONTENTS

CHAPTER ONE: WHAT THIS BOOK WILL DO FOR YOU

To maintain a healthy diet it is important to have all the facts and to know what you can do to help your own overall health. It all begins with developing healthy eating habits. One of the best ways is to eat a wide variety of foods. Simple and easy to follow recipes are pivotal in a successful healthy lifestyle, and one that will you stick with. You need to ensure your body gets the necessary vitamins, minerals and other essential nutrients.

Practicing sports is also another important aspect in maintaining your overall healthy lifestyle. Balancing healthy eating habits and sports, you will maintain healthy body weight and muscle strength. The sport doesn't have to be intense, even moderate intensity physical activities can be beneficial. Some of them activities include: walking, swimming, cycling, hiking, golfing, jogging, bowling, soccer, dancing, or volleyball. For a healthy diet, any activity should be done for at least 30 minutes every day.

Carb cycling has simple ideas that help people in the real world obtain results. Many people have read books, magazines or journals about health and fitness. There is an endless list of dieting plans and some of the common ones include: paleo diets, cabbage soup diet, high protein diets, Atkins, and many more. All these diets come with their own benefits and weaknesses.

With carb cycling, one on the perks is able to enjoy the foods you like and also reduce body fat and weight in the process. This diet is used by athletes, body builders who want to lose weight and fat, stay healthy and keep fit. This book is ideal for you because it will:

a) Provide details about the concept of carb cycling and by following it, you will notice how the diet can and will work.

b) Explain the most important exercises you can incorporate with carb cycling.

c) Assist you in preparing appropriately and give you a fighting chance.

d) Provide a list of foods you must eat and should not eat. It will allow you to have a weekly "cheat meal."

e) Provide you with an action plan you can follow and achieve desired results.

f) Provide a number of recipes.

CHAPTER TWO: ALL ABOUT CARB CYCLING

In this chapter we will discuss carb cycling, and all there is to this unique body-health practice.

There are a lot of definitions that individuals have formulated to explain this particular technique of maintaining a strong and healthy body. Carb cycling is more than just a diet or exercise plan. It is more complex than that. Multiple researchers and enthusiasts talk about and practice Carb cycling respectively, without even understanding what it takes to achieve proper results from this technique.

The term "carb cycling" originates from a diet referred by physicians as CKD, cyclic ketogenic diet. Refers to the consumption of different levels of carbohydrates over different periods of time. The "carb" bit obviously refers to the dietary manipulation of carbohydrates.

But as opposed to whatever explanation you might refer to online, from pages like Wikipedia or other Google search results; this practice has a more diverse connotation. It is more than just a diet, and it entails more procedures than the usual high-intensity exercises. It is not just about food and exercise.

It is quite unsettling to see experts and devotees rely on misconceptions when discussing this practice, especially since it is gaining popularity. Most content that interested researchers find, particularly on this practice, is usually obstructive if not unbecoming.

If you ask me what carb Cycling is, I would tell you that it is too complex of a practice to be phrased in a single sentence. I would rather explain in detail all that it entails.

Carb Cycling Processes

Before you decide to start any carb-cycling process, it is important to know what your short-term and long-term

5

goals are. Do not just start a process without knowing what you want to get out of it; whether it is to build muscles, lose body weight, body health purposes, improve sexual drive, etc.

In this Chapter we will learn the different methods available to suit varying objectives and individuals.

Beginners Guide to Carb-Cycling

After reading so many articles online concerning CarbCycling, I noticed that there are multiple misconceptions that people (professionals and enthusiasts) have about eating meals with low levels of carbohydrates on a daily basis, in order to trim down body fat while maintaining body muscle.

My main concern with this ideology is that having a low-carb or none at all diet, will only be effective over a short period of time. This is because the process will slowly reduce your energy levels and entire body strength. I have to advise my readers that this is not the best way to go about carb cycling, especially if you are trying to maintain your body muscle mass while trimming general body fat.

There is another theory that you have probably read from other books; a confusing illusion that high carb diets are the best and most effective alternatives for weight loss, since they increase the rate of your metabolism. Honestly, these ridiculous theories are far from the truth when it comes to reducing fat. Realistically, there is no single sufficient calorie deficit plan that will assist you to lose weight.

Since neither a low carbohydrate diet nor a high carbohydrate diet will be effective on its own, carb cycling usually helps mitigate the shortcomings of both diets to produce a striking and healthy balance between the two diets, especially if it is done correctly. Carb cycling is a low-carb or no-carb diet that is particularly specific, with intermittent periods where individuals are required to partake in medium or high carbohydrate consumption. For beginners, they are essentially required to alternate their carb intake to realize the preferred effect. Also, for all newfangled folks who practice carb cycling, this particular form of dieting will assist them to maintain their body strength and endure strenuous workouts. Ultimately it will help beginners to experience more positive results.

How to carb cycle: A beginner's guide

A common practice that many beginners choose to do when embarking on carb cycling is to rotate high carbohydrate and low or no carbohydrate days equally throughout the week. However, what most individuals do not realize is that you should do this rotation depending on the goals you have set and your body type. These rotations have to be adjusted and set specifically to suit your needs.

For example, if you are just beginning this practice, you might want to try five low carb days followed by one high carb day. You have to understand that there is no specific set-up that will be appropriate at first, and you will need to tweak your carb days depending on the way your body responds to the carb diet. If you do not do this, it will be difficult for you to realize your specific goals.

Generally, the best way to go about this rotation is by choosing to opt for high carb intake during the days with heaviest training, so as to help support the energy used during those sessions. Low carb days will then be best suited for days with less intense training or no training, otherwise referred to as rest days.

Protein, carbs and fats ratio to follow

I know by now some of you might be wondering about the specific ratio to follow so that you can attain the best outcome. Every individual has diverse macro necessities. This is usually based on the total energy that an individual spends on a daily basis; some books refer this to as TDEE (Total Daily Energy Expenditure). The TDEE of individuals varies due to a number of factors like diet, sex, age, weight, activity levels, lean mass, exercise, physiological state and even hormones.

The weekly ratios that I have suggested below are based on regular strategies. You will be required to adjust these ratios to fit your own needs. If you find this difficult, you can decide to use the standard ratios that I have stated below, in order to match them to your individual requirements, based on what your goals are.

The ratios used below are calculated by multiplying your bodyweight (pounds) times the numbers provided. In order to calculate the total calorie consumption for protein, fats and carbs, simply multiply this value times four (4) for protein and carbs, and times nine (9) for fats.

Carb-Cycling for weight loss

In this section we are going to discuss several techniques, cycles and also the common mistakes that individuals make when trying to lose weight by practicing carb-cycling.

I'm sure you now understand that carb cycling is not only about the diet nor about timeline. You can safely carb cycle your whole life with ease and still remain healthy. There are usually no restrictions with carb cycling. This means that you can gobble up anything from dairy to fruits, from wheat to any other type of macronutrient sustenance. Another added advantage of carb cycling is the positive psychological effect experienced by many people.

To develop a successful carb cycling diet that will help you lose weight, you will have to pay attention to a number of the critical components stated below:

a) You will be required to have a working plan.

b) You will be required to burn more calories than you eat.

c) You will be required to get out of your own way.

When your diet restricts carbohydrates, i.e. low carbs, it is effective in helping individuals lose weight. When you go several days with low carb intake of 50g or less, it eventually causes glycogen levels to drop so low that the body is forced to switch to another fuel resource. You might have heard about this metabolic shift. Professionals refer to it as ketosis. It usually means that the body primarily uses fat as its source of fuel.

Many individuals have decided to adapt this type of lifestyle, and it is not surprising to hear some of these individuals credit a low carb diet for saving their health, if not life. Individuals who are carb cycling enthusiasts tend to follow this diet on a yearly basis, in order to maintain a healthy body weight. Unfortunately, for athletes and those individuals who train intensely, this type of diet is not very practical, especially for individuals who engage in heavy weight training. Eating carbohydrates refills the glycogen in the body and helps the muscles perform at optimum levels.

The dilemma associated with low carb eating is the difficulty experienced in exercise performance, but it is remarkable for weight loss.

Several professionals have tried to formulate different solutions to carb cycling, so that it may give the best result for both worlds. You slowly lower your carbs over a few days. For example, you can start with 190g-200g of carbs then reduce to 110g-120g carbs the following day then reduce to 40g-50g on the 3rd day. You can repeat the cycle from the fourth day or reverse the cycle. When practicing this diet, it is recommended to do intense training on the days that you are consuming high carbohydrates and this should be done after the work out session. This will ensure that the glucose goes directly to your liver and muscles instead of being stored in the body as fat.

Most of the carbcycling diet plans try to incorporate a "cheat day." This particular day is when you are allowed to eat what you want. However, most individuals abuse this day. You should not have more than one "cheat day," and you should maintain consistency throughout the cycle. You have to keep in mind that all successful carb diets are based on a negative calorie balance, especially when individuals use more calories than they consume. Carb cycling does not have a "secret formula." To be able to get around it, you simply have to stick to a single dietary strategy that you find useful.

Common Mistakes That Individuals Make When Trying To Lose Weight through Carb Cycling

1) <u>You are always stressed</u>

So many enthusiasts practice carb cycling with the wrong mental state. You will not realize the full potential of this diet by just eating healthy sustenance or exercising regularly. You are required to make sure that your body is functioning at the most optimum state and that your hormonal environment also favors the whole process. When you get stressed all the time, you end up keeping your body in a constant state of either fight or flight. This usually affects the body by elevating the levels of stress hormones in the body. The most common hormone is the cortisol hormone, which often increases your hunger and cravings, especially for unhealthy foods. Fortunately, this guide will help you to cut back on the stress that you may be experiencing. Try meditation and deep inhalation workout. Ensure that you cut back on online distractions, especially media and social websites. Alternatively, you can try to read books to reduce your stress levels.

What to keep in mind at all times: Chronic stress has a negative effect on your body's hormonal environment. It ends up making you feel hungrier and prevents you from losing weight.

2) __Not cutting back on carbohydrates__

Some individuals respond better to more carbs, as compared to others. Therefore, if you are consuming low-carbs, your weight might stagnate at the same point, so you may want to reduce the carb consumption even further. For example, you can decide to go under 50g of carbohydrates on a daily basis. In order to go under 50g of carbs per day, you will be required to eliminate most fruits from your diet. However, you can decide to eat some berries, but only in small amounts. If this does not work, you can go even further, under 20g. You can continue eating healthy fats, protein and leafy green vegetables. Always ensure that you are eating lowcarb. In addition, you are required to create a free account, especially on the days that you intend to keep fit. Be sure to log your food intake over a period of time.

__What to keep in mind at all times:__ If you notice that you are a carb sensitive individual, then you should eliminate fruits temporarily and eat less than 50g of carbohydrates on a daily basis.

3) __Not consuming appropriate food__

When you decide to practice carb cycling, and in that process decide to follow a lowcarb diet, you have to understand that this process requires more than just lowering your consumption of carbohydrates. You are required to replace those carbs with food that is full of nutrition. Avoid eating low carb foods that have been processed artificially. Processed carbs are fake food products that are NOT suitable for your general health. Carb cycling enthusiasts should stick to fish, meats, eggs, healthy fats and vegetables in order to lose weight.

Another misconception is about the advantages of using "treats," like the ones encouraged from paleo diets. These treats will cause weight problems as much as they are prepared with healthy ingredients. Consider them only as occasional treats and not food that can be consumed on a daily basis.

An important factor is that you should not forget is to eat enough healthy fat. If you decide to cut back on healthy fat and carbs, you will eventually end up feeling very hungry and tired.

When you decide to follow a diet that is not diverse but filled with protein options you will be spoiling yourself and this is an awful idea. Blending high fat with low-carb or mixing moderate proteins with highfat is the way to go, especially if you want to get into ketosis.

What to keep in mind at all times: That you are required to replace the carb options in your diet with real food that is full of nutrition. In order to lose body weight, you will have to stick to eating fish, meats, vegetables and healthy fats.

4) <u>Inadequate sleeping and resting hours</u>

As much as you might not realize it, sleep plays a major role for an individual's overall health. Several studies have shown that when individuals lack sleep it can lead to the development of obesity and weight gain. Also, when you lack sleep you can experience hunger. In addition, you will feel less motivated and generally tired. Even if you are observing proper carb cycling guidelines, you will not achieve proper results if you are not getting proper rest from sleeping.

When you begin carb cycling and working out, most will sleep well. Some individuals do experience sleepless nights or insomnia. You can try some of these tips to improve your sleeping predicament:

a) Ensure that you sleep in complete darkness.

b) Avoid drinking caffeine after two in the afternoon.

c) Try going to bed at a similar time every night.

d) Do something relaxing before you go to sleep, i.e. meditating, deep breathing or reading a book.

e) Avoid drinking alcohol the last few hours before going to sleep.

Refrain from strenuous physical exercise at least 4 hours before going to sleep. *What to keep in mind at all times:* That sleep is of crucial importance in order to achieve optimal health.

5) Wrong exercising techniques or no exercising at all

A common mistake that individuals make when practicing carb cycling is exercising with an objective of burning calories. What they do not know is that the calories actually burned will be insignificant, especially if you consume extra food later on. However, it is important to note that exercise is crucial for both mental and physical health. Doing exercise will help you lose some weight in the long run, and improve your body's metabolic state. It is important to do the correct exercises. I have listed some general exercises and you can expect from doing them with carb cycling.

a) **Interval training** – When you are doing HIIT's (High Intensity Interval Training) you will be improving your cardio health and ultimately your body metabolism. This will raise the levels of human growth hormone in your body.

b) **Weight lifting** – It will greatly enhance the hormonal environment in your body. It will increase your muscle mass. This will help you lose your general body weight in the long term.

c) **Low intensity** – When you do LIIT's (Low Intensity Interval Training) you will always remain active, especially if you try doing something like walking. The human body is naturally designed to move.

What to keep in mind at all times: That the right exercise will ultimately improve your body's hormonal environment. It will also increase your body's muscle mass and you will experience remarkable changes in your body. Mistakes that you should try to avoid include:

- Consuming A lot of Calories
- Eating Too Many Nuts
- Having more than one Cheat day
- Consuming Too Many Sweeteners

Carb Cycling for Body Building and Strength training

In this section we will discuss how carb cycling can help individuals increase their body strength and build muscles at the same time.

In order to achieve these objectives you will be required to balance your intake of carbs. This can prove to be as tricky as trying to balance cardio and strength training. You will be required to consume a lot of carbohydrate meals when training and this usually leaves you with a risk of increasing body fat. Although carbohydrates tend to supply the body with energy. That's why you probably hear or see runners eating lots of pasta before a race.

Since you are not actually expected to exercise every day, you need to understand the importance of nutrients intake. Many science studies have shown that the body has the ability to assimilate nutrients better at particular times of the day. At different time periods you can decide to consume high quantity of carbs without having to increase the fat in your body. Body builders usually require extra calories for strength while training. The most appropriate time to consume carbs is just after a workout or a highly intense sport activity. This is because after strenuous exercise the body's strength is used up, and the muscles are exhausted. This is the appropriate time to have a snack, a meal or a drink that is high in carbs so that the body replenishes energy after the work out.

Many people dream about having a muscular/ripped physique like body builders. Unfortunately when most guys are trying to achieve this goal, they tend to bulk a lot of mass and their muscles fade in the mass gained. When this happens, it is imperative that you develop a way to shred the excess mass. So many times people find themselves at this crossroad, they cannot accept to lose all the mass that they have worked so hard to gain, by dieting down. I refer to this type of individual as "hard gainer."They are also usually resistant to reducing calories.

If you are a hard gainer, you should understand that with carb cycling you can build body mass and lose body fat simultaneously. There are so many articles, from professionals and the inexperienced, on matters concerning this particular concept. I am sure by now many individuals have given up trying to sift through all the information on this subject, especially from the ones who say that you have to choose between the two options, that this concept is not possible.

With this concise guide, you will get the best plan to help you reach this ultimate goal. The guidelines included here are to assist you to not only keep your mass, but to also build your body muscle while burning body fat. Talk about killing three birds with a single stone. In order to achieve this goal, you will be required to demonstrate the upmost discipline.

1) **Consume the right amounts**

Among the most vital points in this plan, is that you need

to eat the appropriate quantities of macronutrients (fats, protein and carbohydrates). By maneuvering these foods and by remaining strict while you are at it, you will start to realize your objective. Carb cycling diet plays a vital role and if you do not adhere to these principles, it will be a waste of your time and energy. You will not achieve your desired physique.

2) **Protein consumption**

Proteins are the main source for building body muscle. Consuming proteins is absolutely necessary, if you are developing a muscle-building strategy. In order to realize your goal, your body requires between 1g to 1.5g of protein per pound of body weight. This means that you will have to consume between 180g-270g of protein, if you weigh 180 pounds. This particular quantity will guarantee that your muscles get the right dose of amino acids, in order to maintain the body's normal metabolic activities and also build the muscle tissues in the body. The most prime protein sources can be found in eggs, chicken, fish, lean steak, turkey, protein powders, ground meat, Greek yogurt and cottage cheese.

3) __Carbohydrates consumption__

Carbohydrates are a great source of muscle energy. You should be mindful of your carbs intake on a day to day basis, to be successful. Be sure to eat meals that consist mainly of fiber and complex carbohydrates. You can find these nutrient combinations in food sources like wild rice, brown rice, wheat pasta, sweet potatoes, some fruits, whole wheat bread and some vegetables.

4) __Fats consumption__

You should never disregard the potential of healthy fats. Specific fats have been regarded to be essential for maintaining certain hormones, like testosterone, which helps the body's energy levels and also increases fat burning in the body. When you consume healthy fats, you will help the body use the fats to replace depleted carbohydrate on the days when your blood sugar levels are down. This will help return the blood sugar level to a more stable level and it will also maintain a steady body health state. Good sources of fats include walnuts, avocado, almonds, olive oil, natural peanut butter, sunflower seeds and egg yolks.

MECHANISMS INVOLVED

For the most crucial part of the procedure, we will look at how to properly manipulate and implement these macronutrients, in order to build strength and muscles, while burning body fat. Although your protein levels will remain the same throughout the process, you will be required to have a constant supply of amino acids for your muscles to recuperate and heal. For starters, you should begin by consuming 1g of protein per pound of bodyweight. Ensure that you continuously assessing your progress. If for some reason you find that you are stalling, you should try to increase the amount to 1.25g or 1.5g per pound. *It is very important that you do not skip this strategy with proteins. It is pivotal in muscle building.*

You will begin to manipulate carbs in a way that your body will be "tricked" into using body fat for fuel. You will consume low carbs for at least two to four days, while the rest of the days will be for medium and high carb food consumption. The explanation behind this reasoning, is that on the days when you consume low carbs, your body will use the fat that is stored for fuel and will leave the muscles alone, as long as the protein intake remains stable. Do not deprive your body of energy. After several days of low carb eating, you will need to consume medium carbs for a day and high carbs the following day.

When you do this, your muscles will have enough fuel to jumpstart your metabolism and there won't be any need to store the body fat, as it will have burned off. An example of carbohydrates intake for a 180 pound person: on low carb days should be 90g, 270g on medium carb days and 405g for high carb days.

Fat consumption should be around 0.25g per pound of bodyweight. However, during low carb days it would be shrewd for individuals to increase their healthy fat intake. This in turn will ensure that hormone levels are kept steady and there will remain enough energy for the intense workouts. What you should consider doing is increasing fat intake by fifty percent on the low carb days. For example, you can eat 3/4 of an avocado on low carb days.

Sample Workout

The routine provided below will enable you to achieve your goals, especially if incorporated with carb cycling:

Key:

RPT- Repetitions

SS- Super S

**Note**: you might want to substitute workouts that you find challenging, but it is discouraged. Also, do not add more exercises to this program, whatever has been presented is enough to help you achieve the desired results. When you are done exercising, you will feel tired and hungry. Indulge in a PWM (post workout meal) that is rich in fats, proteins and carbs.

Carb Cycling for lean physique (Bikini competitions and runners)

The common denominator about both groups of individuals mentioned above is that they both require a body type that is lean in order to suit their respective careers.

You will be surprised at the number of professional runners and bikini models practicing carb cycling. In this section we will discuss how you can practice carb cycling, in order to achieve a lean body, whether it is for running or for competing as a bikini model.

A common mistake that you should avoid making is thinking you are loading up on carbs, when you will be supplying your body with fats.

For both of these careers, maintaining or losing body weight is usually the main point of concern. For runners, this regime involves a bit more planning and being food conscientious, so that it does not interfere with the ability to run. What usually helps individuals in these separate careers to lose weight is calorie deficit. In order to achieve this, individuals are encouraged to control the quality of foods they consume; to be more specific they are discouraged from consuming simple carbohydrates. Alternatively, they are encouraged to eat lowcarb diets, which are more effective.

Runners need to eat a sizable quantity of fuels and calories that contain complex carbohydrates in order to train intensely and to recover as fast as possible from difficult workouts.

If a runner decides to transform or modify the bodybuilding strategy that we discussed earlier, they can attain the delicate balance of the specific metabolic and training demands required from them. They can split the carb cycle process to concur the energy demands required for distance sprinting. Runners are advised to employ different carb cycling methodology that corresponds with specific exercising days. By using this approach, they will be able to target days when calories and carbohydrates are needed for proper performance and recovery. It will also lead to carbohydrate and calorie deficit required for losing body weight.

CHAPTER THREE: CARB CYCLING QUICK-START PROGRAM

The right diet is very important when it comes to building muscle and reducing fat. By putting into practice a few nutritional strategies, you will discover the best way of imitating the effects of anabolic steroids. The nutritional tactics you implement won't take effect immediately and it won't duplicate the effects of anabolic steroids but it will improve your general health and fitness. The nutritional tactics that you should incorporate into your daily life is called, *John O'Malley Carb Cycling Anabolic Environment (JOCCAE)*.

In this book, there has been thorough research and data compiled with the aim of helping people realize that it is possible to build muscle and lose fat at the same time.

Carb cycling is gaining popularity and is considered to be one of the best existing anabolic diets. You need to have a plan. Be committed. Apply this process wisely. Balance it with proper workouts. Understand also that carb cycling without exercising is still effective to maintain your muscle mass and burn fat simultaneously.

John O'Malley Carb Cycling Anabolic Environment (JOCCAE)

You may ask yourself, "why is the John O'Malley Carb Cycling Anabolic Environment (JOCCAE) the best?" "How does it produce better muscle gains?" Well, according to me, I have been using this regime and consider it to be natural, safe and the best way that one can increase muscle building (anabolic) hormones in the body and it is in the same way that steroids do. This diet program will naturally increase your body's production of anabolic hormones, like growth hormone, testosterone and insulin-like growth factor.

This diet program will also help you to have timed and

controlled insulin spikes and this will allow your body to have elevated levels of insulin and growth hormone simultaneously. In normal circumstances this does not happen, but after using this program you will see remarkable muscle gain.

Causes of Muscle Growth

Muscle hypertrophy can be driven by exercising and also excess calories. To encourage muscle growth, you must eat more calories than you use up. Most health experts recommend eating high carb and low fat diets or eating everything in sight, if you want to increase muscle gain. It is important not to assume things because for a child to grow they should not eat more calories, high carb or low fat diets but growth hormones must be released. And as the growth hormones increase they will make the child want to, or start eating more. The purpose of the nutritional strategy in this book is to help you increase the release of anabolic hormones. This guide will help you to know how much to eat and when to eat.

We can build muscle by making ourselves hungry. Instead of using excess calories to help in muscle growth, try to use anabolic hormones, which will increase your appetite to provide enough protein and calories.

John O'Malley Carb Cycling Anabolic Environment (JOCCAE) Diet Breakdown

The diet plan requires you to eat high fat, high protein, low carbohydrate for 5 to 6 days then you carb up for 36 hours. The part of high fat and high protein of the diet is what ignites the increase in the levels of blood serum of growth hormone, testosterone and insulin-like growth factor.

Adaptation of fat

For most of the week, when you will be keeping the level of carbohydrates low, your body will become a machine of fat burning. It will experience a shift in metabolism and start burning fat as its main source of energy. This can take 2 days, but for some people it can take up to 10 days. By the end of the first 5 to 6 days, most will have developed an adaptation to fat. The advantages of fat adaptation include:-

a) Lipolysis (fat breakdown) will increase.

b) Lipogenesis (fat production) will reduce.

c) Catabolism (muscle protein is protected from breakdown) is reduced.

Insulin

First of all, insulin is not anybody's enemy and low carb dieters normally avoid spikes in the levels of insulin. To some, a controlled spike will do you good. Use between 32 to 36 hours, e.g., a weekend, to purposely increase insulin levels. If you don't control insulin levels, it can decrease lipolysis and make you fat. Fat metabolism is regulated by insulin, huge amounts means fat stores for energy will not be given up by your body; the openings to your stored body fat is literally shut, ensuring that no fat is to be released and used for energy. Through a carb loading period, you can increase insulin with the added benefit of:

a) Protein synthesis in skeletal muscle is increased.

b) Helps amino acids to be transported into the muscle

cells.

c) Super-compensation of glycogen (refill muscle glycogen to energize workouts).

Relationship between Insulin and Growth Hormone

I previously stated that increasing growth hormone, insulin and testosterone at the same time will help you to reap the anabolic effects. Normally, when there is an increase in insulin levels the others will decrease and vice versa. Once the body adapts to fat and you continue taking high carbs over 32 – 36 hours, the body will treat it as a threatening condition, and in turn release growth hormone as a survival mechanism. Increasing growth hormones is the best way your body can mobilize energy stores to control this stressful condition and at this time you can get increased growth hormone and insulin at the same time; this will help in muscle gain.

Traditional High Carb (Muscle Building) Diets

When on a high carb diet, the insulin levels are elevated. You can't get the edge of the highest release of growth hormone, fat-gut testosterone and insulin-like growth factor. Also when on high carb diet, you prevent the body from using body fat for energy and in reality, support the laying down of body fat that is new and increased lipogenesis and decreased lipolysis. This anabolic nutritional strategy takes advantage of the anabolic features of insulin and simultaneously controls the hormone's flattening properties. This diet will also help in keeping insulin levels constant and low most of the time, but it is important to keep in mind that you will be generating cautiously timed spikes that will help in muscle growth.

Carbohydrate Threshold Level

Carbohydrate threshold level can be defined as the lowest possible daily intake of carbohydrate that let you to function at peak level. The best thing about this diet is that it can easily fit in your unique type of metabolism. It will help you to find the carbohydrate threshold level and this will allow losing fat without letting go of the lean mass and help in building muscle without fat.

Since our main objective is to gain muscle, we should find the lowest amount of carbohydrates that you need in a day to beat out muscle-gaining exercises that steadily improves. Begin with 30 grams per day then start adjusting from there. You should not make any adjustments to this for at least 6 days because there is a need to make the metabolic change to burning fat for energy first. Once this is finished, you will be able to determine if you need more carbs or not from your exercise performance, if you need more carbs increase by 5 grams per day and keep on checking your weekly averages.

Amount of Carbs, Protein, Fat and Calories to Eat

Many people find it complicated to make decisions on how much and what they are going to eat. This nutritional strategy is all about reducing fat, building muscle.

a) **Step 1:** If you have already confirmed that you will be taking 28 grams of carbs per day then this will come to 112 calories (which is calculated as 27 x 4 calories per gram=112 calories).

b) **Step 2:** You can use a protein calculator to find out how much calories and proteins you need per day. Before using the protein calculator you need to know your current body fat percent and weight. If you eat too much you will definitely get fat. The requirement to build maximum muscle is 200 - 300 calories above maintenance.

> ***Lean Muscle Mass in Kg*** = {Weight in Kg - (Weight in Kg x Body fat (BF) in %)}
>
> ***Protein*** = {2.75 x Lean Muscle Mass in Kg}.
>
> For example, if you are weighing 70 kilograms and your body fat is 40%

then:

Lean Muscle Mass in Kg = {70 - (70 x 0.4)} = 42, and

Protein = {2.75 x 42} = 116.

c) **Step 3:** For you to get the amount of calories you will acquire from protein by multiplying 4 by the grams e.g. 300g = 1200 calories.

d) **Step 4:** Take the combination of carb calories and protein then subtract them from the total calories. For example total cals 2900 - (1200+ 116) = 1584 Calories remaining.

e) **Step 5:** The 1584 Calories will come from dietary fat and if you want to get it in grams divide the figure by 9 and this is mainly because in a gram of fat there are 9 calories. 1584/9 = 176 g fat.

f) **Step 6:** On weekdays, John O'Malley Carb Cycling Anabolic Environment (JOCCAE) is a low-carb, high fat diet. In the above example this person will eat 176 g fat, 116 g protein and 27 g carbohydrate.

Carb-Up Period

After being so strict throughout the week, this is the best period to enjoy life. You decide what to have and whatever you feel like eating, e.g., Chinese food, pizza, and snacks. You can also go out with friends or with your partner and have some drinks while relaxing and enjoying yourself. Because there is no limit on the amount of carbs one can take, you can take as much carbs as you can. The most important thing is to watch how long it takes for you to start to smooth out (loose meaning) at first, it may take a little bit of testing and it will not be the same for everyone. You should therefore not count your carbs or calories during the weekend but relax and enjoy yourself.

You will note that each week you will be going through a small cycle of being smaller and bigger; this is because of variation in water levels. When you start to low carb, some water will be flushed out and this is absolutely normal and natural. You should always keep an eye on your body fat levels in conjunction with your weight. If you observe that by Saturday daylight you are a little bit too much smoothing out, then you know that your carb period should be limited to 24 hours. Keep on observing and making the appropriate changes where necessary.

The John O'Malley Carb Cycling Anabolic Environment (JOCCAE) diet plan is clearly explained for you to understand and put into practice every detail you have learnt. Try eating this way and experience the awesome results it can have on your body.

I have spent a number of months preparing this book for you and I hope you have enjoyed the nutritional strategy diet plan. If you want the most out of this diet and you are looking for a training program, I have created cutting-edge bodyweight training, all backed by science that will help you to build a model's body without even leaving your house. Workouts can help one to build muscles, have incredible strength and it can also help in fat loss.

CHAPTER FOUR: SHOPPING LIST

As you already know carb cycling is an eating plan that involves changing high carb and low carb days. Carb cycling has reward meals that you can eat on a daily basis. It all depends on the plan you are following. This means that you can still eat foods you love, and become healthy and look good. Though there are different plans and they alternate the high carb and low carb days, they do work basically the same each day:

a) You should eat 5 meals a day (do not reduce or increase).

b) Choose foods that are on the shopping list.

c) Drink plenty of water.

For you to lose weight, your body needs the right combination of carbs, healthy fat and proteins and below is the reason you need them:

- **Carbs** are the ideal energy source for your organs and muscles, and they come with those that are healthy and those which are not healthy. The healthy ones include legumes, vegetables, grains and fruits while those which are not healthy include soda, cakes, candy, doughnuts, cookies and other processed foods. Healthy carbs are very important for burning calories and they also help in keeping the energy levels and blood sugar steady.

- **Healthy fats** also known as unsaturated fats when moderately eaten can help the growth and function of your brain and eyes. They can help prevent arthritis, heart disease, depression and stroke. They also keep you from feeling hungry and keep your energy levels stable.

- **Protein** builds and sustains muscles and these muscles help to burn calories. It also breaks down slower than fat and carbs, and this helps it to burn

45

more calories and in turn you will feel fuller longer.
The main reason for alternating high carb and low carb
days in carb cycling is because during the high carb days
you will be stocking calorie-burning heating system so that
during the low carb days your heating system burns lots of
fat. Your metabolism will be tricked by this pattern and it
will be burning a lot of calories, even during the low carb
days.

The best choice for weight loss is a low carb diet, and it
can be combined with a carb up period to be more effective
and simple to maintain. Carb cycling is becoming more
popular because you are allowed to eat cheat foods and still
be able to lose weight faster.
Carb cycling comes with many benefits and some of them
include:

a) It can fit any lifestyle.

b) You are allowed to eat the foods you love.

c) It will help you lose weight and body fat.

d) It will help you to have more energy and feel better.

e) You will be motivated emotionally, physically, spiritually and mentally.

f) It will help you build lean and have strong muscle.

g) Carb cycling also controls hormones concerned with hunger and allows your body to repair its muscle glycogen stores, glycogen is usually important for exercise.

LIST OF FOODS TO EAT

As I explained earlier, you should eat five meals per day. Make sure you eat similar sized portions for each snack or meal. After waking up, eat breakfast within 30 minutes then another snack or meal every 3 hours, for a total of 5 meals per day. Feeding your body keeps your body fueled.

An example of eating times:

- 7 am breakfast
- 10 am snack
- 1 pm lunch
- 4 pm snack
- 7 pm dinner.

Proteins which are lean and have low-sodium

- **Beef:** low-sodium roast beef, cube steak, extra leanground beef, extra leansirloin steak, leanflank steak and round steak.

- **Poultry:** skinless chicken thighs, skinless chicken breast, ground chicken breast, duck breast, low-sodium deli turkey breast, skinless (and not deli) turkey breast and 100% fat-free ground turkey.

- **Game meats:** elk and venison

- **Pork:** low-sodium ham and tenderloin.

- **Shellfish:** clams, lobster and shrimp.

- **Fish:** branzino, cod, grouper, halibut, snapper, Pollock, salmon, sole, sea bass, swordfish, tilefish, tuna, tilapia, trout, catfish, haddock, sardines and flounder.

- **Powdered protein:** rice protein, whey protein, soy protein, egg protein and hemp protein.

- **Dairy:** egg whites, egg substitutes, non-fat plain Greek yogurt and cottage cheese.

- **Vegetable protein:** textured vegetable protein, tempeh and tofu. If you are a vegetarian, the best substitute for any meal is tofu.

Fats

- **Dairy cheeses:** egg yolk, blue cheese, mozzarella, cream cheese, feta cheese, Romano, goat cheese, parmesan, brie, sliced cheeses e.g., gouda, cheddar, Monterey jack, Colby, Havarti, Swiss and muenster.

- **Other dairy:** cream and sour cream.

- **Fruit:** avocado and olives

- **Dressings:** mayonnaise and creamy dressing.

- **Nuts and seeds:** sunflower seeds, almonds, peanut butter, walnuts, almond butter pecans, sesame butter and sesame seeds.

- **Oils:** olive oil and flaxseed oil.

Vegetables

- **Unstarched vegetables:** cabbage, artichokes, rhubarb, snow peas, asparagus, mushrooms, chard, bell peppers, broccoli, broccoli rabe, okra, bok choy, cauliflower, spinach, garlic, collard greens, onions, cucumber, endive, eggplant, fennel, sprouts, wax beans/green beans, radicchio, kale, brussel sprouts, celery, leeks, turnips, mustard greens, peppers, parsley, radishes, salad greens e.g., romaine, arugula and other lettuces, green onions/scallions, shallots, squash, tomatoes and zucchini.

Flavorings

- **Herbs**: including thyme, basil, rosemary and parsley.
- **Spices:** including Cajun seasoning, cayenne pepper, cumin, fennel seeds, garlic powder, ginger, Italian seasoning, paprika, steak seasoning
- Lemon juice, butter spray, chili sauce, marinara sauce, hummus, horseradish sauce, lime juice, tomato sauce, chili paste, salsa, vinegar e.g., white-wine, red-wine, and cider, mustard, hot sauce e.g., Tabasco, low-sodium ketchup, low-sodium broth,

low-sodium soy sauce, tomato paste,low-sodium Worcestershire sauce, extracts e.g., peppermint, almond and vanilla.

- **Salad dressings:** consider one that has fat content; balsamic vinaigrette, Italian dressing and French dressing.

- **Sweeteners:** xylitol e.g., Xylosweet and Xlearstevia e.g., Truvia and Sweet-Leaf, sorbitol, honey in very small amounts and erythritol.

Beverages

- Unsweetened almond milk and unsweetened soy milk.

- Pure coconut water.

- Tomato juice.

- Regular, herbal or green tea.

- Coffee.

- Sparkling or flat Water.

LIST OF FOODS TO LIMIT

The list of foods you should limit, can be eaten on low carb days for breakfast, and in every meal of high carb days.

Fruits

These fruits include; apricots, melons, bananas, pineapple, berries e.g., cherries, blackberries, raspberries, blueberries, and strawberries, mangos, limes, papayas, grapes, apples, grapefruit, peaches, lemons, oranges, nectarines, pears, plums, tangerines and kiwifruit.

Carbs

- **Breads:** brown rice tortillas, Ezekiel 4.9 English muffin, Ezekiel 4.9 breads, Ezekiel 4.9 tortillas, whole-grain bread and corn tortillas.

- **Cereal:** all Bran, low-fat granola, steel-cut oatmeal, Fiber One, old-fashioned oatmeal, Kashi Go Lean, Kashi Heart to Heart and Kashi Good Friends Cereal.

- **Grains:** bran, amaranth, brown rice, wild rice,

barley, popcorn, buckwheat, oats, quinoa and millet.

- **Legumes:** low-sodium canned or boiled beans, lentils, edamame/soybeans and slightly salted soy nuts.
- **Pasta:** couscous, brown rice pasta and whole grain pasta.
- **Root vegetables:** parsnips, yams/sweet potatoes, rutabagas, beets, potatoes and carrots,
- **Starchy vegetables:** peas and corn.

Meal replacement shakes

Contain carbs, vitamins, protein, fiber, and minerals. For no-carb meals avoid shakes that contain carbs.

LIST OF FOODS TO AVOID

These may be eaten in your cheat meals or reward meals/days, but try to keep them out of your kitchen to avoid temptation.

Processed and refined carbohydrates

- Table sugar and other sugars like corn syrup, brown sugar and raw sugar.
- Fruit juice.
- Chocolate, candy, soda with sugar and ice cream.
- White flour/refined flour and any foods that contain it.
- Baked goods such as cookies, bagels, pretzels, crackers, white bread, cake, donuts and pastries.
- White rice and chips.

Processed foods

If you have to get any processed food, look for the low-sodium options.

Fatty foods

- Hydrogenated oils.
- Fried foods.

Foods high in sodium

Alcoholic drinks

- Hard liquor, beer and wine.

Artificial sweeteners

Artificial sweeteners include Saccharin, sucralose, aspartame etc. This will be important when you are cutting back on sugary foods that are processed and getting used to eating whole and healthy food. It is a great idea to go for natural sweeteners rather than artificial ones.

CHAPTER FIVE: CARB CYCLING RECIPES FOR HIGH CARB DAYS

Below is a list of my favorite high carb recipes and they are categorized into dessert, breakfast, lunch and dinner.

BREAKFAST

Greek Yogurt Berry Parfait

Servings: 1

Ingredients:

- 1 cup non-fat plain Greek yogurt
- ½ cup strawberries, sliced
- 2 Tablespoons non-fat granola
- ½ Banana, sliced
- Natural sweetener e.g., Stevia (to taste)

Directions:

1. Combine non-fat plain yogurt with natural sweetener.

2. In a glass parfait dish/mug, layer with Greek yogurt, bananas and strawberries. Repeat until you use up the yogurt.

3. Sprinkle granola over the top and chill for 1 – 2 hours, then serve.

Banana Cream Pie Oatmeal

Servings: 4

Ingredients:

- 1 cup almond milk or low-fat milk
- ¼ cup coconut milk
- ½ cup large flake oats (old fashioned)
- ¼ cup water
- 1 scoop vanilla protein
- ½ banana, sliced

Directions:

1. In a medium saucepan, combine the almond milk and coconut milk, bring to a boil.

2. Add the oats and reduce the heat to medium-low. Stir until milk gets absorbed.

3. In a separate bowl, mix the protein with the water. Stir until completely combined.

4. Pour the oatmeal in a bowl. Pour the protein mixture over the oatmeal. Top with sliced bananas. Serve hot.

LUNCH

Spaghetti Squash with Meat Sauce

Servings: 4

Ingredients:

- 1 Tablespoon melted butter or coconut oil
- 1 large squash(4 cups cooked)
- 2 pinches cinnamon
- 2 pinches salt, 2 pinches pepper (for the squash)
- 1 pound extra lean ground beef
- 2 cups tomato sauce
- 1 Tablespoon olive oil
- 1 cup onion, diced
- ½ cup green pepper, diced
- 1 teaspoon garlic, minced
- 1 teaspoon oregano
- ¼ teaspoon chili powder
- dash of salt, dash of pepper (for the meat sauce)
- ½ cup grated parmesan cheese

- 1 green onion, chopped

Directions:

Preheat oven to 350°F

1. Split the squash carefully. Scrape out the seeds. Drizzle melted butter or coconut oil, salt, pepper and cinnamon over the opened sides of the squash. Place it open-side down in a deep baking dish and fill with water until the opening of the squash is covered. Cover with aluminum foil.

2. Place the dish in the oven. Cook approximately 45 minutes or until the skin can be forked away easily. (If you are unable to cut open the squash, you can cook it whole. Fill a large baking dish to the halfway point with water. Add 15 – 25 minutes cooking time).

3. At the halfway cooking point of the squash. In a large skillet, drizzle olive oil over the bottom, add the diced onion, minced garlic and chopped green pepper. Sweat the vegetables for 5 minutes. Add the

ground beef, cook until completely brown.

4. Once the meat is cooked, add the tomato sauce, oregano, chili powder, salt and pepper. Stir thoroughly. Let it simmer on low while the squash is cooking.

5. Once the squash is cooked, scrape the squash gently with a fork. It will come away stringy. Spoon it into 4 servings.

6. Cover with meat sauce. Top with chopped green onion and grated parmesan cheese. Serve hot. Enjoy!

Turkey Tacos

Servings: 4

Ingredients:

- ½ pound extra lean ground turkey
- 4 yellow or blue corn taco shells
- 1 small onion, diced
- 1 cup shredded lettuce
- ½ cup diced tomato
- ½ cup diced avocado
- dash of salt, dash of pepper
- 2 Tablespoons taco seasoning /or 1 teaspoon chili powder
- ¼ cup water
- ½ cup shredded mozzarella cheese or sharp cheddar cheese

Directions:
Preheat oven to 325°F

1. Place the taco shells on a cookie sheet, and heat

them for 12 – 15 minutes.

2. In a medium frying pan, coat the bottom of the pan with olive oil, add the diced onion. Sweat for 3 – 5 minutes.

3. Add the ground turkey, and dash of salt and dash of pepper, break it up and cook until brown all the way through. Mix the taco seasoning with water. Either add the taco seasoning or chili powder at this point. Mix thoroughly. Cook for another few minutes until the water evaporates and the seasoning is completely combined with the meat.

4. Assemble your tacos. Meat first. Veggies. Cheese. Serve hot. Enjoy!

DINNER

Pesto Chicken Pizza

Servings: 4

Ingredients:

- 1, 6 ounce (approx. ¾ cup) skinless, boneless chicken breast
- dash of salt , dash of pepper
- 2 whole wheat tortilla shells or whole wheat pita
- 3 Tablespoons pesto
- ¼ sundried tomato, thinly sliced
- ¼ cup small broccoli florets
- ½ cup asparagus, cut in bite-sized pieces
- ½ cup aged white cheddar cheese

For cooking pizza in the oven: Recommend using a cast-iron skillet OR a pizza-specific pan, or bake directly on the oven rack. Do not use a cookie sheet as the tortilla or pita won't get crispy.

Directions:

Preheat oven to 400°F

1. Season the chicken breast with salt and pepper. Use your own method to sautée. After cooked, slice the chicken breast into bite-size pieces.

2. Spread the pesto evenly over the tortilla/pita shells.

3. Assemble your pizza: sundried tomato, broccoli, asparagus, chicken. Top with cheese.

4. Place the tortilla or pita directly on the top rack or skillet/pizza pan in the oven. Cook until cheese melts and the tortilla is lightly toasted. Serve hot. Enjoy!

Fruity Chicken Skewers

Servings: 2

Ingredients:

- Bamboo skewer sticks
- 6 ounce skinless, boneless chicken breast, cut in 1 inch cubes
- Fresh pineapple, cut in 1-inch cubes
- Apple, peeled, seeded and cut in 1-inch cubes
- Red pepper, cut in 1 inch chunks
- Onion, cut in 1 inch chunks
- 1 Tablespoon melted butter
- ¼ teaspoon salt
- ½ teaspoon ginger
- ¼ teaspoon chili powder

Directions:

Preheat oven to 350°F

Before you begin to cut up the chicken and vegetables, place the bamboo skewers in water.

1. Everything should be cut into 1-inch cubes.

2. (chicken, pineapple, apple, red pepper and onion)

3. In a bowl mix together the melted butter, salt, ginger and chili powder.

4. Assemble the skewers: Chicken, fruit, onion, red pepper. Repeat.

5. Place the finished skewers in a glass baking dish. Baste the skewers with the marinade.

6. Cook for 12 – 15 minutes. Re-baste with any left-over marinade at the halfway point. Serve hot. Enjoy!

DESSERT

Piña Colada Shake

Servings: 3

Ingredients:

- 1 scoop vanilla whey protein
- 1 Tablespoon shredded coconut
- ½ cup vanilla almond milk
- ½ banana
- ½ cup pineapple chunks
- 1 cup water
- 1 cup ice

Directions:

1. Place the water, ice and almond milk into the blender. Blend until the ice is crushed.

2. Add the banana, shredded coconut, pineapple, and vanilla whey powder. Blend until thoroughly combined. Drink immediately. Enjoy!

Protein Potato

Servings: 2

Ingredients:

- 1 large potato
- 1 cup non-fat cottage cheese
- 2 Tablespoons salsa
- 1 Tablespoon chives

Directions:

1. Bake or steam the potato until soft.

2. Cut the potato in half. Scoop out the middle of the potato.

3. Fill the hollowed out middle with cottage cheese, then salsa. Top with chives. Serve hot. Enjoy!

CHAPTER SIX: CARB CYCLING RECIPE FOR LOW CARB DAYS

Below is a list of some of my favorite low carb recipes suggestions.

BREAKFAST

One Skillet Bacon And Eggs

Servings: 4

Ingredients:

- 8 slices of bacon
- 4 large eggs
- 1 Tablespoon butter
- 1 carrot, peeled and chopped
- ½ cup celery, finely chopped
- ½ white onion, chopped
- ½ cup cauliflower or broccoli, chopped
- ½ cup Colby jack cheese, shredded

Directions:

1. Cut the bacon through the grain into little strips.

2. In a large pan over medium heat, melt the butter. Add the bacon and vegetables.

3. Sauté the vegetables and bacon in the butter for about 15 to 20 minutes, stirring often, until the

71

bacon begins to crisp and the vegetables start to caramelize.

4. Spread the mixture out in the skillet, and create a well in each quarter section.

5. Break an egg into each well. Cover and cook until the eggs are cooked.

6. When the eggs are almost cooked, spread the shredded cheese on top. Continue to cook until the cheese melts. Serve hot. Enjoy!

Bacon Hash

Servings: 2

Ingredients:

- 6 slices of bacon
- 4 eggs
- 1 small onion, chopped
- 1 small pepper, chopped
- few slices of jalapenos (seeds removed)

Directions:

1. Slice the onions and pepper into thin strips. Cut the jalapeno into very small pieces.
2. Cut the bacon into 1 - 2 inch chunks.
3. In a lightly-greased skillet, sauté the vegetables until they become soft. Pour them into a bowl. Set aside.
4. Using a food processor. Pulse the bacon gently. Don't overdo it- just break it up into smaller pieces. (It should not turn into paste-like texture).
5. Add the bacon to the bowl with the vegetables. Mix well.

73

6. Return the vegetables and bacon to the skillet. (You could use egg rings to form the hash when you start cooking. Note: might fall apart when you flip over, keep cooking). Cook the hash until the bacon becomes crispy.

7. You can use the same pan after the hash is cooked to fry the eggs; or cook them in a separate pan as the hash cooks.

8. Scoop the cooked mixture onto a plate. Top with fried egg. Serve hot. Enjoy!

Scrambled Eggs with Ricotta

Servings: 2

Ingredients:

- 2 large eggs
- 1 teaspoon rosemary
- 1 Tablespoon olive oil
- ¾ ricotta cheese, 2% fat content
- ¼ cup Italian salami
- dash of salt, dash of pepper

Directions:

1. Dice the salami into small cubes. In a small skillet, heat the olive oil and fry the salami until golden around the edges.

2. While salami is cooking, in a small bowl, beat the eggs, salt & pepper, and rosemary.

3. Add the ricotta to egg mixture; continue mixing with a fork to break up any lumps.

4. Pour the egg/ricotta mixture into the skillet with the salami. Mix thoroughly. Cook for 5 minutes or until the eggs are fluffy and not shiny. Serve hot. Enjoy!

Crispy Fried Cheddar

Servings: 3

Ingredients:

- ¼ cup cheddar, sliced
- 1 large egg
- 1 Tablespoon olive oil
- 1 teaspoon hemp nuts
- 1 teaspoon ground flaxseed
- 1 teaspoon almond flour (found in most health food stores)
- dash of salt, dash of pepper

Directions:

1. In a bowl, combine the ground flaxseed, hemp nuts and almond flour.

2. Beat the egg, adding salt and pepper.

3. In a medium-sized skillet, heat the olive oil over medium heat.

4. Dip the cheddar slice (one at a time) in the egg mixture, then dip in the dry mixture.

5. Fry for 3 minutes on each side. Serve hot. Enjoy!

Keto Breakfast Muffins

Servings: 9

Ingredients:

- 2 cups ground pork sausage
- 10 large eggs
- 3 cups heavy whipped cream
- 1 cup sharp cheddar cheese, grated or shredded
- 13 cherry tomatoes
- ¾ cup white onion, diced
- ¾ cup green peppers, diced
- 2 ½ cups spinach
- 1 teaspoon garlic powder
- 1 teaspoon onion powder
- dash of salt, dash of pepper
- Muffin pan or silicone muffin cups

Directions:

Preheat oven to 350°F

1. Place frozen spinach in a microwave-safe bowl. Microwave on vegetable mode. Once thawed, place

the spinach in a strainer and press a heavy bowl against the spinach to get rid of any excess liquid.

2. In a separate bowl, break up the ground pork sausage.

3. Dice the peppers and onions. Fry them in a skillet until softened.

4. In another bowl; beat the eggs, add the whipped cream, salt, garlic powder, onion powder, black pepper. Mix until completely combined.

5. Add the egg mixture to the ground pork sausage mixture. Combine thoroughly.

6. Pour the mixture into lightly greased muffin cups or silicone muffin cups. (Note: silicone muffin cups-easier removal of cooked muffin).

7. Optional: add a cherry tomato on top of each muffin cup.

8. Bake muffins for 30 minutes or until they become firm. Serve warm. Enjoy!

Store in an airtight container.

LUNCH

Cheesy Sausage Balls

Servings: 12

Ingredients:

- 12 medium or sharp cheddar cheese cubes
- 1 ½ cups ground sausage, fresh
- ¾ cup mild or medium cheddar cheese, shredded
- Cookie sheet

Directions:

Preheat oven to 400°F

1. Combine the shredded cheese and sausage.

2. Divide the mixture into 12 equal parts.

3. Press a cube of cheese into the center of the sausage mixture. Roll to form a ball.

4. Cover a cookie sheet with aluminum foil. (Note: as oven cooking temps vary and based on a small to medium size sausage ball).

5. Bake the sausage balls for approximately 15 - 20 minutes, or until the sausage is browned.

Serve hot. Enjoy!

Optional: Freeze the sausage balls to use at a later time.

Curry Chicken with Riced Cauliflower

Servings: 6

Ingredients:

- 2 pounds boneless, skinless chicken breasts, raw
- 3 Tablespoons butter
- 1 cup water
- 1 head cauliflower
- 1 packet of curry paste
- ½ cup heavy cream

Directions:

1. Dice the chicken into cubes. Set aside.
2. In a large saucepan, melt the butter. Add the curry paste. Mix well.
3. Once the curry and butter are blended. Add the water. Simmer for 5 minutes.
4. When the liquid mixture is at a steady simmer, add the chicken.
5. Cover the pan with a lid. Let it simmer on a steady boil for 20 minutes.

6. While the chicken is cooking. Dice the cauliflower into florets (remove outer leaves and cut away the core/base). Place the florets in a food processor, pulse gently to break the cauliflower down to a rice consistency. The cauliflower does not need to be cooked.

7. After 20 minutes of cooking the chicken, add the cream and stir. Cook for another 5 minutes without the lid.

8. In the bottom of a bowl, add approximately two (2) scoops of the riced cauliflower. Top with the curry chicken. Serve hot. Enjoy!

Keto Pita Pizza

Servings: 2

Ingredients:

- 14 slices pepperoni
- 1 low-carb pita
- ½ cup Rao's homemade tomato basil marinara sauce

  (can be purchased at Target, Walmart or Amazon)
- ¼ cup grated cheddar cheese
- ⅛ cup (roasted or softened in a pan) red pepper

Directions:

Preheat oven to 425°F

1. Slice the red peppers into strips. Sautée in a pan until softened.

2. Gently separate the pita into 2 pieces. Place on a foil-lined oven pan.

3. Spread a thin layer of olive oil over surface of open pita. Heat in oven 1 - 2 minutes.

4. Pull pan from the oven. Spread marinara sauce over the toasted pita.

5. Spread grated cheese over the pita. Top with the pepperoni and peppers. Place back in the oven. Cook for 5 minutes or until the cheese melts.

Serve hot. Enjoy!

DINNER

Soda Can Burgers

Servings: 5

Ingredients:

- 4 pounds lean ground beef
- 10 slices bacon
- ½ cup extra-sharp cheddar cheese, grated or shredded
- ½ cup pepper jack cheese, cubed
- ¾ cup sliced mushrooms, cooked
- ¾ cup sliced Brussel sprouts, cooked
- ¾ cup sliced green peppers, cooked
- ¾ cup sliced onions, cooked

Directions:

Preheat the grill to 300°F and arrange for indirect heat.

To smoke the meat; use a smoker box or create your own aluminum foil pouch (place a handful of soaked wood chips on a square of foil, wrap the foil tightly around the chips, using a fork, poke a row of holes down the middle). Place the smoker box or wood chips over the ignited burner.

1. Divide the ground beef into even-sized portions. Roll each portion into a large ball.

2. Optional: A light cooking oil rubbed /sprayed around the can- can ease extraction of the can after forming the meat around it.

3. Place the ball of meat onto a hard surface. Place the soda can (or any beverage can) against the middle of the meat and 'smush' (push) the can down.

4. Using your hand, form the meat around the soda can. Push it evenly around and up the can- it should reach about the half-way mark- but will depend on the size of ball of meat you started with. Just make sure the meat is evenly, but not too thinly, distributed around the can.

5. Wrap 2 pieces of bacon around the base of the meat.

6. Remove the can gently.

7. Now you can fill it with the remaining ingredients:

cooked mushrooms, cooked Brussel sprouts, cooked green peppers, and cooked onions.

8. Add the cubed pepper jack cheese on top of the vegetables. Then top with the shredded extra-sharp cheddar cheese.

9. Place each meat patty on the grill - on the side that is not directly heated. Lower the lid and cook for 60 minutes. Any 'smoker' knows you don't lift the lid repeatedly during cooking. You may feel the urge to open the lid but resist *unless* you see flames sprouting! The constant and consistent heat is required to ensure an evenly cooked meat.

10. Cook: 60 minutes = medium-rare; 75 – 90 minutes = well done. Smack the meat in a bun and add your favorite condiments. Serve hot. Enjoy!

Portobello Pizza

Servings: 3

Ingredients:

- 12 pepperoni slices
- 9 spinach leaves
- 3 teaspoons pizza seasoning
- 3 Portobello mushrooms
- 3 slices tomato
- ¼ cup mozzarella cheese, shredded
- ¼ cup cheddar cheese, shredded
- ¼ cup Monterey Jack cheese, shredded
- olive oil, for drizzling
- Cookie sheet

Directions:

Preheat oven to 450°F

1. Remove the stems and wash the mushrooms.

2. Place the mushrooms cap down on a foil-covered cookie sheet/pan. Drizzle olive oil over the mushrooms.

3. Sprinkle pizza seasoning over the mushrooms. Layer a slice of tomato and spinach in the mushroom cap. Spread shredded cheeses over the mushrooms. Sprinkle more pizza seasoning over the cheese.

4. Bake in the oven for 5 minutes, or until the cheese melts.

5. Pull the pan out of the oven. Place slices of pepperoni over the cheese. Pop back in the oven. Cook until pepperoni becomes crispy. Serve hot. Enjoy!

Crockpot Chorizo and Chicken Soup

Servings: 8

Ingredients:

- 4 pounds boneless, skinless chicken thighs, raw
- 4 cups chicken stock
- 1 pound chorizo
- 1 can stewed tomatoes
- 1 cup heavy cream
- 2 Tablespoons garlic, minced
- 2 Tablespoons frank's red hot sauce
- 2 Tablespoons Worcestershire sauce
- Toppings: couple spoonful's of sour cream. Shaved parmesan

Directions:

1. In a non-stick pan, fry the chorizo until brown.
2. In a crockpot- layer the raw chicken thighs then browned chorizo. Add the remaining ingredients: chicken stock, stewed tomatoes, garlic, heavy cream, franks red hot sauce, Worcestershire sauce.

3. Cover and cook on high for 3 hours.

4. After 3 hours, remove the thighs and separate into bite-size pieces. Return the chicken to the crockpot. Cook on low for an additional 30 minutes. Serve hot. Enjoy!

Optional: a dollop of sour cream and shaved parmesan.

DESSERT

Atkins Frozen Coffee

Servings: 6

Ingredients:
- 1 teaspoon vanilla extract
- 3 teaspoons Splenda
- 1 ¾ cup brewed Coffee with water
- 1 cup double cream

Directions:
1. In a medium bowl, mix the brewed coffee and sweetener. Pour into ice cube trays. Freeze the cubes.
2. In a separate bowl, whip the cream. Add the vanilla extract. Then, refrigerate.
3. Get the coffee cubes and put them in the blender to make a slush.
4. Mix the slushy ice cubes with the whipped mixture. Serve cold. Enjoy!

Atkins Chocolate Sundae

Servings: 1

Ingredients:

- 60 gram Atkins' decadent chocolate bar
- 2 Tablespoons non-fat whipped cream
- 2 Tablespoons double cream
- 1 teaspoon Xylitol sweetener, or equivalent sweetener
- 5 Tablespoons almond milk, unsweetened
- ½ teaspoon iodized salt
- 1 teaspoon vanilla extract

Directions:

1. Mix the almond milk, vanilla extract, and double cream in a bowl. Add sweetener and salt. Whisk the ingredients thoroughly.

2. Pour it into an ice cream maker and process according to the manufacturer's instructions. While the ice cream is in the freezer, put your glass bowl

and beaters in the freezer (for whipping whip cream).

3. Once the ice cream has set, just before removing it from the freezer, whip the whip cream, chop the chocolate bar into bite-size pieces. Assemble your sundae: Ice cream, chocolate bits and top with whipped cream.

CHAPTER SEVEN: CARB CYCLING MEAL PLAN

The following is a summary of Meal plans you can adopt for specific carb cycling strategies:

MEAL PLAN 1

Monday- High Carb

- **Breakfast:** Scrambled egg white, one cup of veggies and toast.

- **1ˢᵗ Nibble:** A pint of chocolate milk, two cups of greens and oats.

- **Lunch:** Cube steak (3 oz.), sweet potatoes and broccoli.

- **2ⁿᵈ Nibble:** A pint of chocolate milk, two cups of greens and oats.

- **Dinner:** Baked tilapia (4 oz.), Mexican slaw and two corn tortillas.

Tuesday- Low Carb/No Carb

- **Breakfast:** Scrambled egg white, one cup of veggies and toast.
- **1ˢᵗ Nibble:** 150g Greek yoghurt, two cups of greens and peanut butter.
- **Lunch:** Cube steak (3 oz.), cheese (1 oz.) and steamed spinach.
- **2ⁿᵈ Nibble:** 150g Greek yoghurt, two cups of greens and peanut butter.
- **Dinner:** One bacon slice, steak (3 oz.) and Brussels sprouts.

Wednesday-High Carb

- **Breakfast:** Scrambled egg white, one cup of veggies and toast.
- **1ˢᵗ Nibble:** A pint of chocolate milk, two cups of greens and oats.

- **Lunch:** Cube steak (3 oz.), sweet potatoes and broccoli.

- **2nd Nibble:** A pint of chocolate milk, two cups of greens and oats.

- **Dinner:** Baked tilapia (4 oz.), Mexican slaw and two corn tortillas.

Thursday-Low Carb

- **Breakfast:** Scrambled egg white, one cup of veggies and toast.

- **1st Nibble:** A pint of chocolate milk, two cups of greens and peanut butter.

- **Lunch:** Baked tilapia (4 oz.), Mexican slaw and quarter Avocado.

- **2nd Nibble:** 150g Greek yoghurt, two cups of greens and peanut butter.

- **Dinner:** One bacon slice, steak (3 oz.) and Brussels sprouts.

Friday-Low Carb/No Carb

- **Breakfast:** Scrambled egg white, one cup of veggies and toast.

- **1ˢᵗ Nibble:** 150g Greek yoghurt, two cups of greens and peanut butter.

- **Lunch:** Cube steak (3 oz.), cheese (1 oz.) and steamed spinach.

- **2ⁿᵈ Nibble:** A pint of chocolate milk, two cups of greens and peanut.

- **Dinner:** Cube steak (3 oz.), cheese (1 oz.) and steamed spinach.

Saturday-High Carb

- **Breakfast:** Scrambled egg white, one cup of veggies and toast

- **1ˢᵗ Nibble:** A pint of chocolate milk, two cups of greens and oats.

- **Lunch:** Turkey patty & tomato, lettuce and baked Potato fries.

- **2ⁿᵈ Nibble:** 150g Greek yoghurt, two cups of greens and oats.

- **Dinner:** Baked tilapia (4 oz.), Mexican slaw and two corn tortillas.

Sunday is a cheat day and you can eat anything you like.

MEAL PLAN 2

Meal 1:

- **High carb:** Porridge, honey, semi skimmed milk, orange juice and bananas.
- **Low carb:** Berries, granola and natural yoghurt.
- **No carb:** A pint of chocolate milk.

Meal 2:

- **High carb:** Crisp bread crackers, cheese, handful of nuts, sultanas and raisins.
- **Low carb:** 150g Greek yoghurt.
- **No carb:** Pineapple and cottage cheese.

Meal 3:

- **High carb:** Banana, salad with mayonnaise and chicken.
- **Low carb:** Tuna salad, whole meal bread and apple.
- **No carb:** Chicken Salad.

Meal 4:

- **High carb:** Apple, flapjack and Progain.

- **Low carb:** Peanut butter and snack-a-jacks.

- **No carb:** Handful of nuts.

Meal 5:

- **High carb:** Natural yoghurt, sweet potato, mushrooms and sirloin steak.

- **Low carb:** Chicken, peanuts, low fat rice and pudding.

- **No carb:** Salmon, Broccoli and Spinach.

Meal 6:

- **High carb:** Peanut butter, skimmed milk and crisp bread.

- **Low carb:** Fruit and natural yoghurt.

- **No carb:** Chicken pieces.

Meal 7:

- **High carb:** A pint of chocolate milk.

- **Low carb:** 150g Greek yoghurt.

- **No carb:** A pint of chocolate milk.

CONCLUSION

I hope this book was able to help you understand everything you needed to know about carb cycling diet and most importantly, it enlightened you on how beneficial it can be for weight loss, muscle building and improving your general health.

The next step is for you to put into practice what you have learned in this book and experience the remarkable effect it can have in your body, and also, on your life.

CHECK OUT OTHER RESOURCES:

All the following books are available on Amazon.

While practicing carb cycling you can also work out. If you are looking for the best workouts that can help you build a model's body without even leaving your house.

I also have 2 other bodyweight training programs, to help you grow a specific muscle group fast:

Calisthenics: 7-Day Chest-Blasting Calisthenics Program To Gain Up To 3 Inches In 7 Days

Calisthenics: 7-Day Arm-Blasting Calisthenics Program To Gain Up To An Inch In 7 Days

94354498R00062

Made in the USA
Middletown, DE
18 October 2018